"Mommy What's AIDS?"

JOYCE NORTHRUP DODGE

Tyndale House Publishers, Inc.
WHEATON, ILLINOIS

Cover and interior illustrations by Mary Beth Schwark

Library of Congress Catalog Card Number 89-50499
ISBN 0-8423-4375-X
Copyright 1989 by Joyce Northrup Dodge
Printed in the United States of America

1 2 3 4 5 6 7 8 9 10 95 94 93 92 91 90 89

Dedicated with love

to the children

of our world

through whom

God passes

his righteousness

from one generation

to another

AIDS is a relatively new disease.
Information about AIDS appears daily in newspapers
and on the television, but most people still have lots of
questions. And children have lots of questions, too.
"Will I get AIDS? Will my friends at school get AIDS?
How do you get AIDS? Do you die from AIDS? Can
you get AIDS if you know someone who has AIDS or
if someone in their family has AIDS? Is there anything I
can do to make sure I don't get AIDS?"

Unfortunately, not all of these questions can be
answered with certainty. But there are many things we
can and must teach our children about AIDS. It is even
more important that we teach them about the type of
life-style God designed us to live: a life-style of sexual
abstinence before marriage and mutual faithfulness in
marriage; a life-style that does not include homosex-
uality or drug use or abuse.

This book is designed for parents to read aloud with

their children. It will give answers to the questions kids are asking about AIDS, and it stresses the absolute importance of following God's plan as outlined in the Bible for the way we should live.

Discussion about AIDS necessarily involves explicit discussion of both heterosexual and homosexual sex, though these discussions are handled sensitively and from a biblical perspective. Also, because of the street language to which our children are exposed, we will use medical terms to add dignity in the explanation of these subjects. It is recommended that parents talk with their children about the basic elements of sexuality before reading this book together. A list of recommended books about sex education is found at the back of this book, as well as a glossary of technical terms used in this book.

*D*ad honked the horn of the car as he drove up to the house. Sally and David ran out of the house and down the front steps to meet him. It was always fun when Dad came home! Dinner and the evening together were happy times in their family.

nine

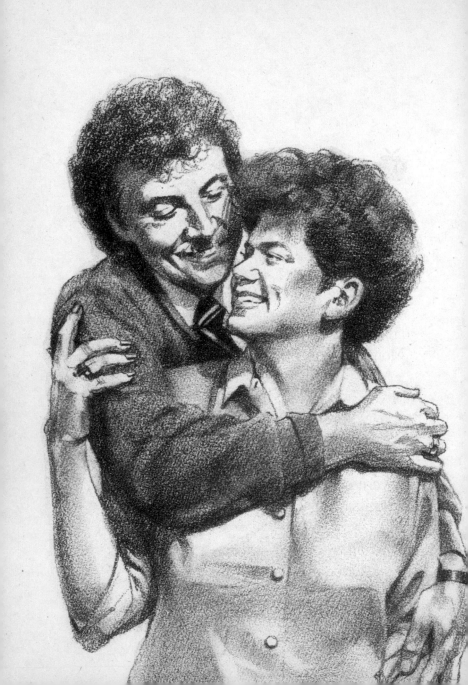

"It smells like good food in here," Dad said as he gave Mom a big hug. "I'm hungry as a bear!"

"I'm glad you're home," Mom said, smiling. "Dinner's all ready."

The family sat at the table, enjoying their dinner and talking. Suddenly David asked, "Mommy, what's AIDS?"

Mom looked at Dad, then at David. "Why do you ask, Son?"

"The kids say that some people don't want my friend Randy to come to school anymore because he has AIDS," David answered with concerned eyes and a worried voice.

"I'm so sorry to hear that, David," Mom said.

"So am I, David," Dad said. "After dinner let's talk about it."

eleven

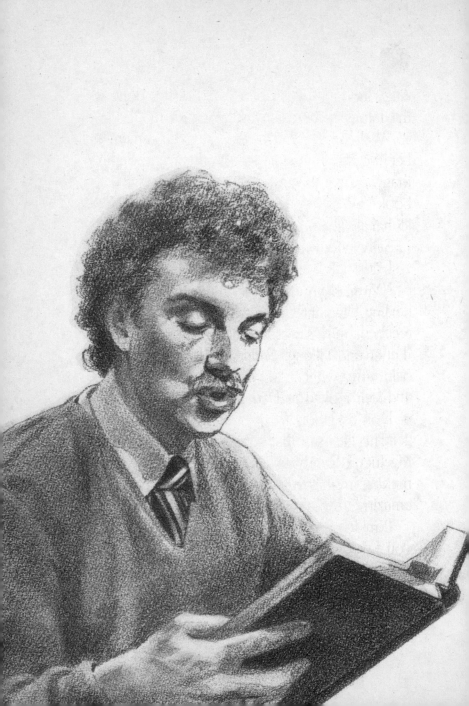

After the table was cleared and dishes done, the family gathered in the living room.

"Well, kids," Dad began, "do you remember the beautiful story of Abraham and Sarah that we read together from your Bible story book? Do you remember how Sarah gave birth to her son, Isaac?"

Sally nodded her head. "I remember."

Dad smiled and said, "That is God's beautiful picture of a family. He wants us to have a family to love and care for us." Dad reached for the Bible on the coffee table. "Let's read from Psalm 139. Perhaps that will help you to understand what AIDS is, David, and help you know how to help your friend."

Dad began to read, "You made all the delicate, inner parts of my body, and knit them together in my mother's womb. Thank you for making me so wonderfully complex! It is amazing to think about."

Looking up from the Bible, Dad asked, "Do you know what that means, kids?"

David and Sally looked at each other, not sure what answer to give.

thirteen

GOD HAS
CREATED
OUR BODIES
IN A
WONDERFUL
WAY.

"God has created our bodies in a wonderful way," Mom explained. "He gave us arms, legs, feet, toes, and other parts that we can see and touch. He made hearts and brains that are inside our bodies."

Dad nodded and added, "God also made some very important openings in our bodies. Each opening has a job to do, as well as something to protect it. If something gets in an opening that doesn't belong there, the body can get infected or sick."

fifteen

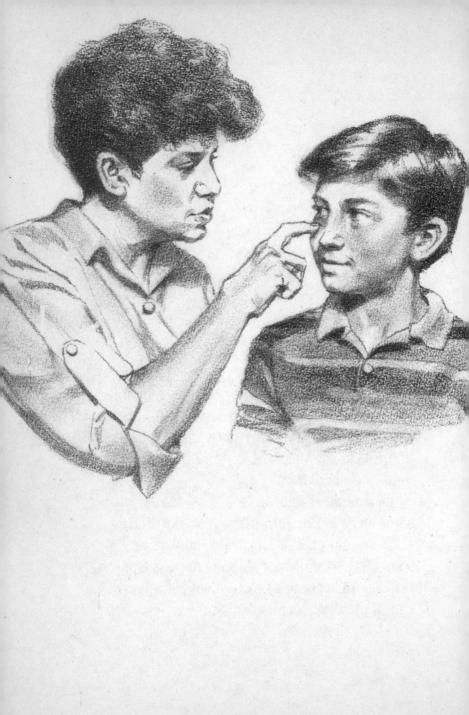

Mom pointed to David's eye. "The job or function of your eye is to see, David. God made the eyelid, the eyebrow, and tears to protect this opening. Do you remember when Uncle Fred got a piece of steel in his eye at his machine shop?"

"I remember," Sally said. "Uncle Fred had to go to the hospital, and a doctor took the piece of steel out of his eye."

David nodded. "Uncle Fred told us that his eye might have gotten infected because that piece of metal was in his eye and it didn't belong there."

seventeen

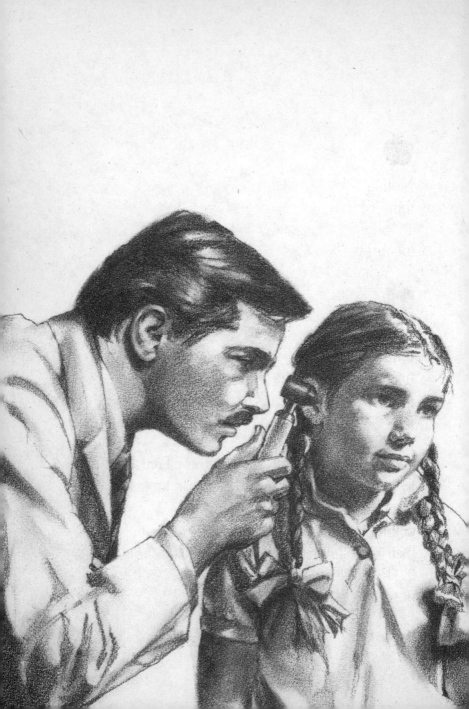

Mother asked another question. "Can you think of another opening in your body?"

"Sure," David said, raising his hand to touch his ear. "My ear is an opening."

"What job does your ear have, David?" Dad asked.

"Hearing," David quickly responded.

Mom smiled. "Do you remember when little Judy next door put a bean in her ear when I was baby-sitting her? We had to take her to the doctor, and he used a long pair of tweezers to take out the bean because it didn't belong in Judy's ear."

"Some other body openings are the nostrils in your nose," Dad said. "And your mouth. And some people have put things that don't belong in these openings—things like beans in their noses or poison in their mouths."

"I sure don't want to get anything in my nose that doesn't belong there," Sally said.

GOD'S PLANS
FOR US
ARE
BEAUTIFUL.

Mom asked, "Do you kids remember when we talked recently about God's beautiful plan for the way babies are born? We told you that girls have a special opening called the vagina. God's plan is that the woman's husband puts his penis in his wife's vagina. When he does this, the husband's sperm comes out of his penis and into his wife's vagina. We call this 'sexual intercourse.'"

Dad looked at his children and spoke in a soft, gentle voice. "If a girl waits until after she is married for sexual intercourse, she is called a virgin. God's plan is for people to have sexual intercourse only after they are married.

"But sometimes people choose not to follow God's perfect plan for sexual intercourse. If they don't follow God's plan, and if they misuse the openings of the body God gave them, their bodies can become infected."

twenty-one

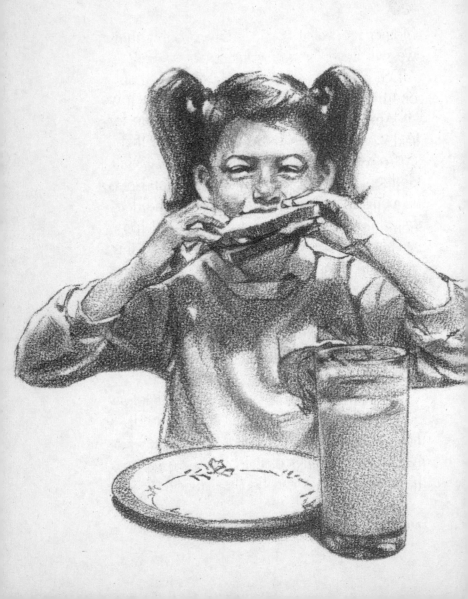

Mother looked at David. "You probably think we will never answer your question about AIDS. But we will, right after we talk about one more opening."

"And about a peanut butter sandwich," Dad said.

"A peanut butter sandwich?" Sally asked, surprised.

Mom smiled at her. "When you come home from school, you always ask for a glass of milk and a peanut butter sandwich."

Dad nodded. "When you eat your sandwich, something marvelous happens. Inside your body are intestines that take valuable things called nutrients from the sandwich. Your body can then use the nutrients to give you energy, to build bones, and to keep you healthy."

Mother continued. "And what is left over from the sandwich is called waste. This waste comes out when you go to the bathroom, as urine and as feces. The intestines get rid of the

IF WASTE
COULD NOT
LEAVE
OUR BODIES,
WE WOULD
GET
VERY SICK.

feces waste by moving it down through the body opening called the anal opening. So the function of the anal opening is to get rid of waste material. If this waste could not leave our bodies, our stomachs would hurt and we would get very sick."

"Our buttocks help protect the anal opening," Dad added. "God has put a very strong muscle there so the waste won't come out too easily and to keep things out that don't belong in the anal opening."

Dad paused for a moment, then continued. "Now children, listen very carefully. When a man is sexually attracted to a woman, and a woman is sexually attracted to a man, they are called heterosexual. They are attracted to the opposite sex.

"But there are people who are sexually attracted to people of the same sex—men to other men, women to other women. These people are called homosexuals. And some

QUESTIONS
ABOUT **AIDS**
ARE NOT
EASY TO
ANSWER.

homosexual men have sexual intercourse by putting their penises into other men's anal openings. When they do this, several bad things can happen. The fragile tissue of the anal opening can be seriously damaged or torn. And one or both of them can get AIDS, which is a very serious disease. When people get AIDS, they get very sick and weak, and then they die.

"And homosexuals are not the only people who can get AIDS. If a homosexual who has AIDS also has sexual intercourse with a woman, she can get AIDS. Then she can pass it on to other men with whom she has sexual intercourse."

David and Sally were very quiet for a moment. "Daddy, how could Randy get AIDS?" David asked. "He isn't a homosexual, and he hasn't had sexual intercourse with anyone."

"Mommy, will I get AIDS?" Sally whispered.

"We'll try to answer your question first, David," Dad said, "and then yours, Sally. Please remember that they are not easy

BLOOD
TRANSFUSIONS
ARE MUCH
SAFER
NOW.

questions to answer because even doctors don't really know all the answers."

Mother nodded and said, "Sexual contact is not the only way AIDS can be passed on. A person can also get AIDS through the exchange of blood by a blood transfusion and possibly by coming in contact with the urine and feces of someone who has AIDS.

"David, your friend Randy was in an accident several years ago and had to have a blood transfusion. Some of the blood in blood banks had the AIDS virus in it and doctors didn't know it. When some sick people, like Randy, were given blood transfusions, they received blood with the AIDS virus. And they became sick with the AIDS disease."

Mom looked at David. "That is very sad. And I'm so sorry this happened to Randy. Doctors now use a test to find the AIDS virus in blood, and this makes blood transfusions much safer."

THE MOST
COMMON
WAY OF
GETTING
AIDS
IS BY
HAVING SEX
WITH
SOMEONE
WHO HAS
AIDS.

"Now for your question, Sally," Dad said. "As far as doctors know, the most common way of getting the AIDS virus is through sexual intercourse with someone who has AIDS. Another common way of spreading AIDS is when people who use drugs use the same hypodermic needles. Also, a woman who has the AIDS virus can pass it on to her unborn baby because the baby receives some of the mother's blood. So babies of drug users and people who have sex with drug users can get AIDS."

DO YOU
SEE HOW
BEAUTIFUL
AND WISE
GOD'S PLANS
ARE?

Mom put her arms around her children. "As far as doctors and scientists know, AIDS is not spread by being near someone who has AIDS, or even from taking care of a person with AIDS. And since the AIDS virus cannot live long outside of the body, doctors and scientists don't believe AIDS is spread by sneezing and coughing, or by sitting on a toilet seat or drinking from a water fountain that was used by someone with AIDS."

Dad smiled tenderly at David and Sally. "Do you see how beautiful and wise God's plans for us are? He wants us to avoid sexual contact before we are married, and he wants us to have sexual intercourse only with our husband or wife. And he wants us to say no to doing things that will hurt our bodies, like the wrong use of drugs.

"Following his plans will bring us much joy

thirty-three

JESUS
WANTS US
TO LOVE
AND
PRAY FOR
PEOPLE
WHO ARE
SICK AND
FRIGHTENED.

and help protect us from many painful consequences, such as AIDS."

"Always remember," Mom said, "that God gives us his plans for us because he loves us very much."

"Mommy, does God love people who have AIDS?" Sally asked.

"Yes, Sally, he does. And he wants *us* to love them, too. He wants us to pray for them and for their families. He wants us to find ways we can help them. He wants us to treat them kindly.

"Some followers of Jesus have opened special houses to help people who are dying from AIDS," Dad said. "Some churches help people who have AIDS by going to clean their houses or cook for them or take them to the doctor. Other people take babies with AIDS into their homes and care for them. All of these people are living the words of Jesus when he said, 'I was sick and you visited me.' Jesus touched people who were sick, even if they had scary diseases like leprosy."

"David, would you like to do something for your friend Randy?" Mom asked. "Would you

GOD
CAN HELP
PEOPLE
WITH
AIDS
NOT TO BE
AFRAID.

like to have him come home with you for cookies and milk and play video games?"

"Oh, yes, Mommy," Randy said. "I would like that."

"Having AIDS is a very frightening and difficult thing," Dad said. "But God can help people with AIDS not to be so afraid. And he can help us not to be afraid of them or their disease, and to love them."

Everyone was silent for a moment. Then Mom and Dad gathered the children into a family circle. They prayed together, thanking God for being a loving Father who cares for us all.

"Thank you, God," Dad prayed, "for being a loving Father who has given us wonderful bodies, and for teaching us ways to care for our bodies. Help us to follow your commands. And help people who have serious diseases. Show us ways we can be kind and reach out to those who are suffering—and share your love with all those around us.

"We love you, God. Amen."

TERMS USED IN THIS BOOK

Anal Opening The outlet of the rectum, the end of the tube that makes up the digestive system. The anal opening lies in the fold between the buttocks.

Feces Body waste such as food residue, bacteria, and mucus moved out of the bowels through the anal opening.

Heterosexual A person who is sexually attracted to persons of the opposite sex.

Homosexual A person who is sexually attracted to persons of the same sex.

Intestines A long tube that extends from the stomach to the lower end of the large intestine. Part of the digestive system.

Penis The male organ used for sexual intercourse and for getting rid of body waste fluids (urine).

Sexual Intercourse Sexual union between a male and a female.

Sperm Cells formed in a part of the male's reproductive organ. When a sperm from a male enters a female's egg, the egg is fertilized. The fertilized egg will then go into a part of the female's body called the uterus and develop into a baby.

Transfusion When one person's blood is put into another person's bloodstream.

Urine A body waste fluid that goes from the cells into the bloodstream. The blood carries the waste to the kidneys, then to the bladder, until it finally leaves the body through a tube called the urethra.

Vagina A small tunnel in a female that leads from the uterus to the outside opening of the genital canal.

Virgin A person who has not had sexual intercourse.

RECOMMENDED READING

Sex Education

Jane Graver, *How You Got to Be You* (St. Louis: Concordia, 1982).

Carol Greene, *Each One Specially* (St. Louis: Concordia, 1982).

Ruth Hummel, *I Wonder Why* (St. Louis: Concordia, 1982).

Kenneth N. Taylor, *Almost Twelve* (Wheaton, Ill.: Tyndale House Publishers, Inc., 1968).

AIDS information

Linda Meeks and Philip Heit, *AIDS: What You Should Know* (Columbus, Ohio: Merrill Publishing Company, 1987). A twenty-seven-page booklet that has student and teacher editions and is designed for use with 6th, 7th, and 8th graders. Presents topically organized information, avoids explicit and detailed discussion of risky sexual practices, and does not address use of condoms; teaches that abstinence is most responsible decision to make regarding both sexual activity and drug use.

Stephen R. Sroka, *Educator's Guide to AIDS and other STD's* (Lakewood, Ohio: Health Education Consultants, 1987). Presents abstinence as the most effective method of preventing AIDS and emphasizes responsible sexual behavior and prevention of drug use.

SUMMARY:
How AIDS Is and Is Not Transmitted

AIDS **is** transmitted by:
1. Having sexual intercourse with someone who has the AIDS virus;
2. Sharing intravenous (IV) drug needles with a person who has the AIDS virus;
3. An unborn child receiving the virus from the mother;
4. Receiving a blood transfusion of infected blood.

AIDS **is not** transmitted by:
1. Casual contact with a person, such as shaking hands, hugging, or social kissing;
2. Sharing food or drinks;
3. Sneezing, coughing, or sweating;
4. Eating out in a restaurant or swimming in a pool;
5. Using public drinking fountains, restrooms, or telephones;
6. Pets or insects;
7. Donating blood.

FOR CHILDREN:
Ways to Avoid Getting AIDS

1. Do not have sex until you are married, and then have sex only with your spouse.

2. Do not use drugs (and don't drink, since alcohol weakens your ability to fight off infections and can affect your judgment, causing you to do unsafe things that you normally might not do).

3. Keep your immune system strong by eating nutritious meals, getting exercise and enough rest, and not smoking.

4. Discuss your fears about AIDS with your parents or with an adult you trust. Don't act out of ignorance; find out the truth about AIDS and how it is transmitted, and act accordingly.

FOR PARENTS:
Ways to Protect Your Children from AIDS

1. Help your children develop clear standards of right and wrong. Children who have a firm grasp of appropriate moral behavior are less likely to engage in behaviors that put them at risk of becoming infected with AIDS. Establish clear and specific standards in your home regarding behavior.

2. Teach sexual abstinence before marriage as a biblical and social virtue. Show the scriptural basis for right and wrong regarding sexual standards and behavior.

3. Establish your family unit as a source of acceptance and support. When your children see the fidelity and commitment you and your spouse have for each other and for your children, they will learn that these traits are positive goals. And it is a fact that uninfected persons in mutually faithful and monogamous relationships are protected from contracting AIDS through sexual transmission.

4. Set a good example. The most effective teacher your children have is your behavior. Treating your spouse according to the scriptural standards of love and fidelity will

go a long way toward teaching your children the proper ways to express love and affection. Also, following standards of good health—a healthy diet, exercise, and so on—will give your children a good example of how to care for themselves and their bodies.

5. Encourage your children not to give in to peer pressure. Help them identify how peer pressure can be a negative influence for them, and help them develop ways to resist this pressure when it comes.

6. Be informed about AIDS, drugs, and alcohol so that you can discuss these topics with your children and provide them with knowledgeable guidance. Stress scriptural guidelines for these areas, too (such as 1 Corinthians 6:19-20 and Romans 14:7-8). When discussing any of these things, present the facts in a straightforward manner and emphasize the biblical standards of right and wrong behaviors. Help your children to understand that God is not trying to be a cosmic killjoy; rather, he has given us guidelines that will lead us into lives that are as happy and healthy as they can be.

LIST OF INFORMATION SOURCES

Toll-Free National Information
The National AIDS Hotline
1-800-342-2437
Operates seven days a week, twenty-four hours a day.
The staff answers questions, refers callers to local and
national hotlines and testing sites, and gives telephone
numbers for counseling, financial aid information, and
support groups. Free written material available on request.

School and Community Resources
AMERICAN RED CROSS
Operates an AIDS Public Education Program for providing
reliable, factual data. Materials include pamphlets and a
four-part AIDS prevention program featuring a videotape
and printed material for junior- and senior-high school
students. Contact local Red Cross chapters or the American
Red Cross, AIDS Education Program, National
Headquarters, 1730 E St., N.W., Washington, DC
20006, (202) 639-3223.

AIDS School Health Education Subfile
A computerized subfile of the Combined Health
Information Database that contains information about
AIDS programs, curricula, guidelines, policies, regulations,
and other materials. Call Bibliographic Retrieval Service
Information Technologies to obtain access to the data
(1-800-468-0908), or write BRS Information
Technologies, 1200 Route 7, Latham, NY 12110.
There is a time charge and a fee for obtaining a password.